EMMANUEL JOSEPH

Mental Health in the Elderly: The mental health challenges faced by the elderly population, especially in long-term care facilities

Contents

1

Chapter 1: Introduction - Understanding the Aging Population and Mental Health

As our population ages, the mental health of our elderly citizens becomes an increasingly critical concern. This chapter serves as the foundation for our exploration of the complex and multifaceted challenges faced by the elderly, particularly those residing in long-term care facilities. It sets the stage for understanding the unique mental health needs of this demographic, the factors contributing to their vulnerabilities, and the importance of addressing these concerns.

The Aging Population: A Global Perspective

The world is experiencing a significant demographic shift. According to the World Health Organization, the number of individuals aged 60 and over is expected to double by 2050, accounting for over 22% of the global population. This aging demographic brings both opportunities and challenges, with mental health being a central concern. Understanding the aging population's mental health needs is crucial to improving their overall well-being and quality of life.

Aging and Mental Health: A Dynamic Interplay

1

Aging is a natural process, and it is associated with a myriad of physical, cognitive, and emotional changes. Some of these changes are normal, such as age-related cognitive decline, while others are related to various mental health issues. It's essential to recognize that aging does not inherently lead to mental health problems, but it can increase vulnerability to specific challenges.

Mental Health Challenges Faced by the Elderly

The elderly population faces a range of mental health challenges, including depression, anxiety, dementia, loneliness, and substance abuse, among others. These challenges can be attributed to various factors, including biological changes, social isolation, loss of loved ones, and the stressors associated with aging.

Long-Term Care Facilities: A Complex Setting

Long-term care facilities, such as nursing homes and assisted living facilities, play a crucial role in providing care for elderly individuals who may require assistance with daily activities or have significant health issues. However, these settings have their unique set of challenges, including potential isolation, institutionalization effects, and inadequate mental health support.

The Importance of Addressing Mental Health in the Elderly

Recognizing and addressing the mental health needs of the elderly is not just a matter of compassion; it is a public health imperative. Untreated mental health issues in this population can lead to diminished quality of life, increased morbidity, and higher healthcare costs. Furthermore, these issues can have far-reaching effects on families and society as a whole.

The Road Ahead

In the chapters that follow, we will delve into the specific mental health challenges that the elderly face, exploring the factors contributing to these challenges and discussing strategies for prevention, intervention, and support. We will also examine the role of caregivers, healthcare professionals, and policymakers in shaping the future of mental healthcare for the aging population.

This introductory chapter sets the stage for a comprehensive examination of mental health in the elderly, highlighting the urgency and importance of addressing these challenges as our world continues to age.

2

Chapter 2: The Aging Brain: Cognitive Changes and Mental Health

As we continue our journey into the world of mental health challenges faced by the elderly, this chapter explores the intricate relationship between cognitive changes and mental health in the aging population. It is essential to understand how these changes impact an individual's emotional and psychological well-being, as they often play a central role in the development and management of mental health issues.

The Aging Brain: A Complex Landscape

Aging brings about a series of neurobiological changes that influence cognitive functions. These changes include alterations in brain structure, neurotransmitter levels, and synaptic plasticity. While some cognitive abilities remain stable, others, such as processing speed and working memory, tend to decline with age. Understanding the dynamics of these changes is fundamental to comprehending their effect on mental health.

Cognitive Reserve and Resilience

Cognitive reserve refers to an individual's ability to optimize or maximize cognitive performance in the presence of age-related brain changes. Factors such as education, mental stimulation, and engagement in challenging activities can enhance cognitive reserve. These factors not only influence cognitive abilities but also play a role in mental health resilience as individuals age.

The Interplay Between Cognitive Changes and Mental Health

Cognitive changes can have a profound impact on mental health in the elderly. Memory decline, difficulty with problem-solving, and cognitive impairments are often linked to increased feelings of frustration, stress, and even depression. It is crucial to recognize the early signs of cognitive decline and their potential consequences on an individual's mental well-being.

Distinguishing Normal Aging from Cognitive Disorders

It's essential to differentiate between normal age-related cognitive changes and cognitive disorders such as Alzheimer's disease or other forms of dementia. While some cognitive decline is considered a part of the aging process, more severe cognitive impairments require medical evaluation and support. Understanding this distinction is vital for timely intervention and treatment.

Promoting Cognitive Health and Mental Well-Being

This chapter also explores strategies and lifestyle choices that can support cognitive health in the elderly. Engaging in mentally stimulating activities, maintaining a healthy diet, and staying socially connected are all associated with better cognitive function and improved mental well-being. We will discuss practical ways to promote cognitive and emotional resilience in later life.

The Role of Caregivers and Healthcare Professionals

Family members, caregivers, and healthcare professionals have a critical role in recognizing cognitive changes and their implications for mental health. Understanding the challenges that cognitive changes bring, along with strategies for communication and support, is vital for providing effective care to the elderly population.

Conclusion

In this chapter, we have established a foundational understanding of the aging brain's cognitive changes and their impact on mental health. As we continue our exploration of mental health in the elderly, we will delve deeper into the specific mental health challenges associated with these cognitive changes and discuss strategies for maintaining and improving mental well-being in the face of cognitive decline.

3

Chapter 3: Depression in the Elderly: A Silent Epidemic

Depression is a prevalent and often under-recognized mental health issue among the elderly. This chapter sheds light on the unique aspects of depression in late life, its causes, risk factors, and the importance of early detection and treatment.

The Prevalence of Depression in the Elderly

Depression affects a significant proportion of the elderly population. It is estimated that approximately 5-10% of older adults experience depressive symptoms, and rates are even higher among those residing in long-term care facilities. Despite its prevalence, depression in the elderly often goes undiagnosed and untreated, earning it the reputation of a "silent epidemic."

Recognizing Depression: Symptoms and Challenges

Depression in the elderly can manifest differently than in younger individuals. Symptoms may include persistent sadness, loss of interest in previously enjoyed activities, changes in appetite and sleep patterns, fatigue, and physical complaints. Distinguishing depressive symptoms from other age-related changes or medical conditions can be challenging but is essential for accurate diagnosis.

Causes and Risk Factors

Understanding the causes and risk factors for late-life depression is vital for both prevention and intervention. Factors such as genetic predisposition, chronic medical conditions, social isolation, and bereavement can contribute to the development of depression in the elderly. The interaction between these factors and an individual's unique life circumstances plays a significant role.

Complications and Consequences

Depression in the elderly is associated with various complications and consequences. These can include impaired physical health, decreased cognitive function, an increased risk of suicide, and a reduced quality of life. The close link between depression and physical health issues emphasizes the importance of integrated care that addresses both mental and physical well-being.

Treatment Approaches and Interventions

Effective treatment of depression in the elderly often involves a combination of psychotherapy, medication, and lifestyle modifications. This chapter discusses evidence-based treatment approaches and highlights the importance of tailoring interventions to the unique needs of older adults. It also explores the challenges of medication management, especially in cases where individuals are taking multiple medications for chronic conditions.

The Role of Caregivers and Support Systems

Caregivers, family members, and healthcare professionals play a crucial role in recognizing and supporting elderly individuals dealing with depression. They can provide emotional support, encourage engagement in meaningful activities, and help facilitate access to professional help. Moreover, building a strong support system can mitigate the impact of depression and improve the overall well-being of the elderly.

Reducing Stigma and Promoting Awareness

Reducing the stigma associated with depression in the elderly is essential for encouraging open conversations and seeking help. This chapter explores strategies for reducing stigma, raising awareness about the importance of mental health in late life, and advocating for improved mental healthcare for the elderly.

Conclusion

Depression is a significant and often overlooked mental health challenge in the elderly population. Understanding its unique features, causes, and consequences is the first step toward better detection, intervention, and support for older adults experiencing depressive symptoms. As we move forward in this book, we will continue to explore other critical mental health issues affecting the elderly and discuss strategies for addressing them in various contexts, including long-term care facilities.

4

Chapter 4: Anxiety Disorders in Late Life

Anxiety disorders are among the most common mental health issues in the elderly, yet they are often overshadowed by other conditions like depression. This chapter focuses on anxiety disorders in late life, their manifestations, causes, and the importance of recognizing and addressing these conditions.

The Prevalence of Anxiety Disorders in the Elderly

Anxiety disorders affect a significant portion of the elderly population, with estimates ranging from 10% to 20% of older adults experiencing symptoms of anxiety. These disorders encompass a wide range of conditions, including generalized anxiety disorder, panic disorder, social anxiety disorder, and specific phobias.

Manifestations and Symptomatology

Anxiety disorders can manifest differently in older adults than in younger individuals. Symptoms may include excessive worry, restlessness, muscle tension, and physical symptoms like heart palpitations or digestive issues. Understanding these manifestations is crucial for timely diagnosis and intervention.

Causes and Risk Factors

The causes of anxiety disorders in late life are multifaceted. They can be triggered by life transitions, such as retirement or the loss of a loved one, as well as by chronic medical conditions and cognitive impairments. Additionally, there may be a genetic predisposition to anxiety that becomes more pronounced with age.

Overlapping Symptoms with Other Conditions

Anxiety disorders in the elderly often co-occur with other medical and psychiatric conditions, including depression and dementia. This overlap can complicate diagnosis and treatment, emphasizing the need for comprehensive assessments and tailored interventions.

Impact on Physical Health

Anxiety disorders can have a significant impact on an individual's physical health, leading to sleep disturbances, high blood pressure, and an increased risk of heart disease. These physical health consequences highlight the interconnectedness of mental and physical well-being in the elderly.

Treatment Approaches and Interventions

This chapter delves into evidence-based treatment approaches for anxiety disorders in late life, such as cognitive-behavioral therapy and medication. It emphasizes the importance of individualized treatment plans that consider the unique needs and preferences of elderly patients.

The Role of Caregivers and Healthcare Professionals

Caregivers and healthcare professionals play a vital role in recognizing and addressing anxiety disorders in the elderly. They can provide emotional support, create a safe and reassuring environment, and help individuals access appropriate treatment and therapy. Additionally, caregivers should be aware of their own mental health and stress levels, as these can impact the person they are caring for.

Strategies for Coping and Prevention

This chapter discusses coping strategies for individuals living with anxiety disorders in late life. It also explores preventive measures, such as stress reduction techniques, regular physical activity, and social engagement, that can help reduce the risk of developing anxiety disorders as one ages.

Conclusion

Anxiety disorders in the elderly are a prevalent and often underdiagnosed mental health issue. Recognizing the unique features and challenges of these conditions is essential for improving the well-being of older adults. As we continue our exploration of mental health in late life, we will address other key issues and provide insights into the support and care needed for the elderly population, particularly in long-term care facilities.

5

Chapter 5: Dementia and Alzheimer's Disease: Impact on Mental Health

Dementia, particularly Alzheimer's disease, is a significant mental health concern in the elderly population. This chapter delves into the profound impact of dementia on mental health, the challenges it poses for individuals and their caregivers, and the strategies for providing quality care.

The Prevalence of Dementia in the Elderly

Dementia is a collective term for a group of cognitive disorders characterized by a decline in memory, thinking, and reasoning abilities. Alzheimer's disease is the most common cause of dementia, affecting millions of individuals worldwide. Understanding the prevalence of these conditions in the elderly is essential for recognizing their impact on mental health.

Cognitive Decline and Emotional Well-Being

Dementia leads to significant cognitive decline, which can result in emotional distress, confusion, and frustration for affected individuals. The inability to remember loved ones, manage daily tasks, and communicate effectively can

13

lead to feelings of sadness, anxiety, and agitation.

Challenges for Caregivers and Families

Family members and caregivers of individuals with dementia often bear a substantial burden. Providing care for those with cognitive impairments can be emotionally and physically taxing. This chapter explores the challenges faced by caregivers and the importance of support systems in helping them cope with the demands of dementia care.

Grief and Loss: A Continuous Process

The progression of dementia and Alzheimer's disease is often marked by a series of losses—loss of memories, abilities, and eventually, the loss of the person as they were known. Coping with this ongoing grief process is a significant aspect of the mental health challenges faced by both individuals with dementia and their loved ones.

Behavioral and Psychological Symptoms of Dementia

This chapter discusses the behavioral and psychological symptoms often seen in dementia, including aggression, agitation, and wandering. Understanding these symptoms is crucial for providing appropriate care and ensuring the safety and well-being of individuals with dementia.

Support and Interventions

Effective strategies and interventions can improve the quality of life for individuals with dementia and support their mental health. This chapter explores non-pharmacological approaches, such as reminiscence therapy and structured routines, as well as medication options for managing behavioral symptoms.

The Importance of Early Diagnosis

Early diagnosis of dementia is crucial for implementing interventions and support systems that can enhance the mental well-being of affected individuals. The chapter discusses the significance of early recognition and the potential benefits of early intervention.

Future Directions in Dementia Care

As research continues to advance, new approaches to dementia care and treatment are emerging. This chapter explores promising avenues in dementia care, including technology-based solutions, caregiver support programs, and person-centered care approaches.

Conclusion

Dementia, particularly Alzheimer's disease, is a formidable challenge that profoundly affects the mental health of the elderly and their caregivers. This chapter provides insights into the emotional toll of dementia and the importance of comprehensive care strategies that address not only the cognitive decline but also the psychological and emotional needs of those affected. As we continue to explore mental health issues in late life, we will consider the broader context of care, including the role of long-term care facilities in supporting individuals with dementia.

6

Chapter 6: Loneliness and Social Isolation: A Growing Concern

L oneliness and social isolation are increasingly recognized as significant mental health challenges faced by the elderly. In this chapter, we delve into the profound impact of these issues on mental well-being, explore their causes, and discuss strategies for combating the loneliness epidemic.

The Loneliness Epidemic

Loneliness is a pervasive issue in the elderly population, with a substantial proportion of older adults reporting feelings of isolation. As people age, they may face changes such as the loss of a spouse, retirement, or physical limitations, which can contribute to a sense of social disconnection.

The Link Between Loneliness and Mental Health

Loneliness is not merely a fleeting emotion; it can have profound and lasting effects on mental health. Persistent loneliness is associated with a higher risk of depression, anxiety, cognitive decline, and even physical health issues such as cardiovascular disease. Understanding the connection between loneliness and mental health is crucial for addressing these issues.

Social Isolation: A Related Challenge

Social isolation, often resulting from a lack of social connections, is closely related to loneliness. It can be exacerbated by factors such as limited mobility, transportation barriers, or a lack of available social opportunities. Social isolation further contributes to feelings of loneliness and negatively impacts mental well-being.

Addressing the Root Causes

This chapter explores the root causes of loneliness and social isolation in the elderly. It considers factors such as bereavement, retirement, living arrangements, and technological barriers that can contribute to these feelings. Recognizing these causes is the first step in developing effective interventions.

Strategies for Combating Loneliness and Social Isolation

The chapter discusses a range of strategies aimed at reducing loneliness and social isolation. These strategies include community programs, senior centers, intergenerational activities, and technology-assisted communication tools. Providing opportunities for social engagement is essential for addressing these challenges.

The Role of Healthcare Professionals

Healthcare professionals play a critical role in recognizing and addressing loneliness and social isolation in the elderly. They can screen for these issues, provide support, and connect individuals to appropriate resources and services. Collaborative efforts with social workers and mental health professionals are essential for a comprehensive approach to care.

Building Social Support Networks

This chapter emphasizes the importance of building social support networks for the elderly. Support from family, friends, and community organizations can significantly reduce feelings of loneliness and isolation. The chapter also highlights the importance of maintaining and nurturing these connections.

Conclusion

Loneliness and social isolation are pervasive issues that profoundly affect the mental health of the elderly. Recognizing and addressing these challenges is vital for improving the overall well-being of older adults. As we continue to explore mental health issues in late life, we will delve into strategies for creating more inclusive and supportive communities, including long-term care facilities, that combat loneliness and foster social engagement.

7

Chapter 7: Substance Abuse and Addiction in Older Adults

Substance abuse and addiction are not limited to the younger population; they are increasingly recognized as critical mental health concerns in older adults. This chapter examines the unique challenges of substance abuse in the elderly, its causes, and strategies for prevention and intervention.

The Hidden Issue of Substance Abuse in the Elderly

Substance abuse and addiction often go unnoticed in older adults. However, the misuse of alcohol, prescription medications, and other substances is a growing concern in this demographic. Understanding the prevalence and patterns of substance abuse in the elderly is the first step in addressing this issue.

Unique Factors Contributing to Substance Abuse

Several unique factors contribute to substance abuse in older adults, including chronic pain, loneliness, retirement, and bereavement. Additionally, older adults may have medications prescribed for various health conditions, making them vulnerable to misuse.

The Impact on Mental Health

Substance abuse can have severe consequences for mental health, exacerbating conditions such as depression and anxiety. It can also lead to cognitive impairments, strained family relationships, and an increased risk of accidents and injuries.

Recognizing Substance Abuse

This chapter discusses the challenges of recognizing substance abuse in older adults, as it often presents differently than in younger individuals. Signs may include changes in appetite, sleep disturbances, neglect of personal hygiene, and memory problems. Effective screening and assessment tools are vital for early detection.

Dual Diagnosis: Co-occurring Mental Health and Substance Use Disorders

It is not uncommon for older adults to experience both mental health issues and substance use disorders simultaneously. This chapter explores the concept of dual diagnosis and the complexities of providing integrated care to address both conditions effectively.

Treatment and Intervention

Effective treatment of substance abuse in the elderly involves a combination of medical, psychological, and social interventions. This chapter discusses evidence-based treatment approaches, such as motivational interviewing and cognitive-behavioral therapy, and highlights the importance of personalized treatment plans.

Preventive Strategies

Prevention is key to addressing substance abuse in older adults. This chapter explores strategies for preventing substance misuse, including education, responsible prescribing practices, and promoting healthy coping mechanisms for age-related challenges.

The Role of Healthcare Professionals

Healthcare professionals, including physicians, nurses, and social workers, play a vital role in recognizing and addressing substance abuse in older adults. They must be trained to assess and intervene when substance misuse is suspected. Collaboration with addiction specialists is often necessary for comprehensive care.

Conclusion

Substance abuse and addiction are complex issues that affect mental health in older adults. Recognizing the signs and symptoms of substance abuse, understanding the unique factors contributing to this problem, and providing effective treatment and prevention strategies are essential for improving the well-being of older adults. As we continue our exploration of mental health issues in late life, we will discuss additional challenges and solutions, particularly within the context of long-term care facilities.

8

Chapter 8: Grief and Bereavement: Coping with Loss in Late Life

Grief and bereavement are natural processes that individuals face throughout their lives, but they take on unique dimensions in late life. This chapter delves into the profound impact of loss on mental health in the elderly, the specific challenges they encounter, and strategies for coping and support.

Grief in Late Life

As people age, they often experience multiple losses, including the death of spouses, friends, and family members. Grief can be a prevalent and ongoing experience in late life. Understanding the unique aspects of grief in this stage of life is essential.

Manifestations of Grief

Grief can manifest differently in the elderly than in younger individuals. Common emotional responses may include sadness, anger, guilt, and feelings of emptiness. Physically, individuals may experience changes in sleep patterns, appetite, and energy levels.

Complicated Grief

Some individuals in late life may experience complicated grief, where their grief response is prolonged, intense, or significantly impairs their ability to function. This chapter explores the risk factors and implications of complicated grief, emphasizing the importance of early intervention.

Loss and Mental Health

Grief can have a significant impact on mental health in late life. It is associated with an increased risk of depression, anxiety, and loneliness. Recognizing this connection between grief and mental health is critical for providing appropriate support and care.

The Role of Culture and Spirituality

Culture and spirituality play a significant role in how individuals cope with loss in late life. This chapter explores the diversity of cultural and spiritual practices related to grief and highlights the importance of respecting and supporting an individual's unique beliefs and traditions.

Coping Strategies and Support

This chapter discusses coping strategies that can help individuals navigate grief and bereavement. It explores the benefits of seeking support from family, friends, and support groups, as well as the potential role of therapy or counseling in the grieving process.

The Grief of Caregivers

In late life, individuals may be both the recipient of care and the caregiver, leading to complex grief dynamics. This chapter examines the unique challenges faced by caregivers when they experience loss and grief in the context of providing care to their loved ones.

Building Resilience in Late Life

Resilience is an essential aspect of coping with grief in late life. This chapter explores strategies for building emotional resilience, finding meaning in loss, and fostering personal growth through the grieving process.

Conclusion

Grief and bereavement are universal experiences that take on unique dimensions in late life. Understanding the impact of grief on mental health, recognizing the challenges faced by the elderly, and providing compassionate support are essential for helping older adults navigate the complex journey of loss. As we continue our exploration of mental health issues in late life, we will discuss further aspects of care and support, including the role of long-term care facilities in addressing these challenges.

9

Chapter 9: Psychosocial Factors in Long-Term Care Facilities

Long-term care facilities, including nursing homes and assisted living centers, play a significant role in the lives of many elderly individuals. This chapter delves into the psychosocial factors that impact mental health in these settings, exploring the challenges and strategies for enhancing the well-being of residents.

The Transition to Long-Term Care

Entering a long-term care facility can be a significant life transition for older adults. This chapter explores the emotional and psychological challenges that residents may face during this transition, including feelings of loss, disorientation, and the need to adapt to a new environment.

Social Integration and Loneliness

Long-term care facilities vary in terms of their social environments. Some residents may experience a sense of community and companionship, while others may grapple with feelings of loneliness and isolation. This chapter discusses the factors that contribute to social integration and the strategies that facilities can employ to foster a sense of belonging.

Quality of Care and Staff Relationships

The quality of care provided by staff in long-term care facilities directly impacts the mental health of residents. The chapter explores the importance of respectful and compassionate care, staff-resident relationships, and effective communication in supporting the emotional well-being of elderly residents.

Emotional Support and Psychological Services

Many elderly residents of long-term care facilities may benefit from emotional support and psychological services. This chapter discusses the role of mental health professionals, such as counselors and psychologists, in addressing the psychosocial needs of residents. It also highlights the importance of emotional support from family and friends.

Activities and Engagement

Engagement in meaningful activities is essential for the mental well-being of elderly residents. The chapter explores the role of structured programs, recreational activities, and creative outlets in promoting a sense of purpose and fulfillment within long-term care settings.

Privacy, Autonomy, and Dignity

Respecting the privacy, autonomy, and dignity of residents is fundamental to their mental health. This chapter discusses the challenges and strategies for preserving these vital aspects of a person's identity and well-being within the institutional setting of long-term care facilities.

Coping with Loss and End-of-Life Care

Grief and loss are a part of life in long-term care facilities, where residents may pass away or experience the loss of friends and acquaintances. This chapter examines the strategies and support needed to cope with loss and provides insights into end-of-life care within these settings.

The Role of Family and Caregivers

Family members and caregivers play a crucial role in supporting the emotional well-being of elderly residents in long-term care. This chapter discusses the dynamics of family involvement, providing practical guidance for families seeking to advocate for their loved ones in these settings.

Conclusion

Long-term care facilities are an integral part of the lives of many elderly individuals, and their psychosocial factors significantly impact residents' mental health. Understanding the challenges faced by residents and the strategies for enhancing well-being within these settings is essential for improving the quality of life for the elderly in long-term care. As we continue our exploration of mental health issues in late life, we will discuss additional topics, including the role of caregivers, therapeutic interventions, and policy considerations.

10

Chapter 10: Caregiver Burnout and Support

Caring for elderly individuals, especially those facing mental health challenges, can significantly impact the well-being of caregivers. This chapter examines the phenomenon of caregiver burnout, its implications, and strategies for providing support to those who provide care for the elderly.

Understanding Caregiver Burnout

Caregiver burnout is a state of physical, emotional, and mental exhaustion resulting from the demands of caregiving. This chapter explores the causes and symptoms of caregiver burnout, including stress, fatigue, feelings of isolation, and a sense of being overwhelmed.

The Impact of Caregiver Burnout

The impact of caregiver burnout extends beyond the individual providing care. It affects the quality of care provided, the caregiver's health, relationships, and overall well-being. This chapter examines the implications of burnout on both the caregiver and the person receiving care.

Recognizing Signs and Coping Strategies

Recognizing the signs of burnout is crucial for preventing its escalation. This chapter discusses strategies for managing stress, setting boundaries, seeking social support, and utilizing self-care practices to prevent and cope with caregiver burnout.

Support Services and Resources

Access to support services and resources can significantly alleviate caregiver burden. The chapter highlights available support networks, respite care options, caregiver support groups, and community resources that provide assistance to caregivers in managing their responsibilities.

Importance of Self-Care for Caregivers

Prioritizing self-care is essential for caregivers to maintain their own well-being while caring for others. This chapter emphasizes the significance of self-care practices, such as regular breaks, engaging in hobbies, seeking professional help, and maintaining a healthy lifestyle.

Building Resilience and Seeking Help

Developing resilience and knowing when to seek help are critical aspects of caregiving. The chapter explores resilience-building strategies and emphasizes the importance of seeking assistance from healthcare professionals or support groups when needed.

Respecting Caregivers' Needs and Rights

Respecting caregivers' needs, rights, and limitations is fundamental. This chapter discusses the importance of recognizing caregivers as partners in care, advocating for their rights, and providing them with the necessary resources and appreciation.

Conclusion: Supporting Caregivers for Better Elderly Care

Caregivers play a pivotal role in the lives of the elderly. This concluding chapter emphasizes the significance of supporting caregivers to ensure the well-being of both the elderly individuals they care for and themselves. It highlights the importance of a holistic approach that values and supports caregivers' mental, emotional, and physical health needs.

This chapter provides insights into understanding, addressing, and preventing caregiver burnout, ultimately promoting a more sustainable and compassionate caregiving environment for the elderly.

11

Chapter 11: Therapeutic Interventions and Treatment Approaches

Therapeutic interventions and treatment approaches are central to addressing mental health challenges in the elderly. This chapter explores the various methods and strategies employed by mental health professionals to support the emotional and psychological well-being of older adults.

Individual Psychotherapy

Individual psychotherapy, including cognitive-behavioral therapy, psychodynamic therapy, and person-centered therapy, can be highly effective in addressing a range of mental health issues in the elderly. This chapter discusses the principles and application of these therapies for older adults.

Group Therapy and Support Groups

Group therapy and support groups provide opportunities for elderly individuals to connect with peers, share experiences, and receive support. This chapter explores the benefits of group interventions, such as reducing feelings of isolation and fostering a sense of community.

Reminiscence Therapy

Reminiscence therapy involves discussing and reflecting on past experiences, which can be a particularly meaningful intervention for the elderly. This chapter delves into the applications of reminiscence therapy for improving mental well-being, enhancing memory, and providing a sense of purpose.

Music and Art Therapy

Music and art therapy offer alternative approaches to traditional talk therapy. This chapter explores the use of creative arts as therapeutic interventions, highlighting their ability to promote self-expression, emotional release, and cognitive stimulation.

Physical Activity and Mind-Body Interventions

Physical activity, yoga, and relaxation techniques play a crucial role in supporting mental health in the elderly. This chapter discusses the benefits of physical and mind-body interventions, such as reducing stress, improving mood, and enhancing overall well-being.

Medication Management

In some cases, medication is a critical component of treating mental health issues in the elderly. This chapter explores the use of medication, the importance of careful medication management, and potential side effects and interactions in older adults.

Telehealth and Technology-Assisted Interventions

Advances in technology have opened new avenues for providing mental health support to the elderly. This chapter discusses the use of telehealth, smartphone applications, and other technological solutions in delivering therapeutic interventions to older adults, even in remote or long-term care settings.

Cultural Competence and Ethical Considerations

Providing therapeutic interventions in late life requires cultural competence and sensitivity to the unique ethical considerations of this population. The chapter explores the importance of respecting cultural diversity and upholding ethical principles in mental health care for the elderly.

Family and Caregiver Involvement

In many cases, family members and caregivers are integral to the success of therapeutic interventions. This chapter discusses the role of family and caregivers in supporting and participating in the treatment process, emphasizing the importance of collaboration and communication.

Conclusion

Therapeutic interventions and treatment approaches are essential components of mental health care for the elderly. Understanding the diverse range of options available, tailoring interventions to individual needs, and considering the involvement of family and caregivers are vital for addressing the unique challenges and opportunities in providing mental health support to older adults. As we continue our exploration of mental health issues in late life, we will also address policy considerations and strategies for promoting resilience and well-being in aging.

12

Chapter 12: Promoting Resilience and Well-Being in Aging

Promoting resilience and well-being in aging is a multifaceted endeavor that encompasses various factors, including physical, mental, and social aspects of life. This final chapter of our book explores strategies and approaches to help elderly individuals lead fulfilling and resilient lives as they age.

Resilience in Aging

Resilience is the ability to adapt and bounce back in the face of adversity, and it is crucial for maintaining well-being in aging. This chapter discusses the importance of cultivating resilience and explores the factors that contribute to resilience in the elderly.

Physical Health and Well-Being

Maintaining physical health is fundamental to well-being in aging. This chapter highlights strategies for staying physically active, adopting a nutritious diet, and engaging in regular health check-ups to support a healthy and active lifestyle.

Cognitive Health and Mental Stimulation

Cognitive health is essential for maintaining mental well-being. The chapter discusses activities and practices that promote cognitive stimulation, such as brain exercises, lifelong learning, and engagement in mentally stimulating hobbies.

Social Engagement and Support

Maintaining social connections and support systems is vital for well-being in aging. This chapter explores the benefits of social engagement, the importance of maintaining meaningful relationships, and strategies for connecting with others, both within and outside long-term care facilities.

Emotional Resilience and Coping Strategies

Developing emotional resilience is crucial for coping with the challenges of aging. The chapter discusses emotional coping strategies, including stress management, mindfulness, and emotional regulation techniques that can help elderly individuals adapt to life changes.

End-of-Life Planning and Advance Directives

End-of-life planning is a crucial aspect of promoting well-being in aging. This chapter addresses the importance of discussing end-of-life wishes, creating advance directives, and ensuring that one's values and preferences are respected as they approach the end of life.

Policy Considerations and Advocacy

Advocacy and policy considerations play a role in shaping the well-being of the elderly. This chapter explores the importance of advocating for supportive policies that address the unique needs of older adults and promote access to quality healthcare and social services.

Lifelong Learning and Personal Growth

Lifelong learning and personal growth are essential components of well-being in aging. The chapter discusses the benefits of pursuing new interests, setting personal goals, and finding purpose and fulfillment in later life.

Spirituality and Finding Meaning

Spirituality and the search for meaning can provide significant support in aging. This chapter explores the role of spirituality in promoting well-being and offers insights into finding meaning in late life.

Conclusion: Embracing Aging with Resilience and Well-Being

Promoting resilience and well-being in aging is a lifelong journey that requires a combination of physical, mental, and social efforts. This concluding chapter encourages readers to embrace the process of aging with resilience and a commitment to maintaining well-being throughout the later years. It also emphasizes the importance of continuing research, awareness, and support for the mental health needs of the elderly population.